Keto in Five

Easy Five Ingredient Keto Diet Recipes With 5 Ingredients or Less & 5 Net Carbs or Less

Introduction

You Are About To Discover How To Make Your Keto Dieting Easy, Affordable, Less Complicated And Highly Effective By Leveraging The Power Of These 5 Ingredient Keto Diet Recipes That Have Net Carbs And Less!

The keto diet is indeed highly effective in switching the body to become an efficient fat burning machine. Its effectiveness is evident based on the sheer number of recipes you will find online for suit all manner of dieters; from vegetarian to vegan to smoothies and much more.

One thing is still a problem though; many times, the fact that the ingredients are too many means that it can be quite costly to prepare keto meals affordably. Moreover, with many ingredients, you can expect the steps to be just as many and complicated. And that's not even the bad part; when you have many ingredients, the chances of having recipes with lots of carbs per serving is very high, which essentially means if you overeat a little, you could actually be innocently getting yourself out of ketosis.

This book is meant to solve just that by having a collection of handpicked keto diet recipes that have 5 ingredients only, that can be prepared in 5 steps only and that yield five servings or less as well as 5 net carbs or less.

With that, you can bet that getting into ketosis and staying in there will be an effortless affair! Some recipes even have zero carbs!

So if you are tired of having to follow long keto diet recipes that use tons ingredients to a point where you feel lost?

Are looking for recipes that are straightforward and less complicated and

Don't want to keep spending a fortune just to follow the keto diet

This book is for you!

In it, you will find delicious five ingredient keto diet recipes with 5 steps or less and yielding 5 servings or less and with 5 net carbs per serving!

You will find recipes for:

- Breakfast
- **Lunch**
- Dinner
- **Dessert**
- Snacks
- And much more

And it is not just a bunch of boring bland recipes; the recipes in here will make you wonder whether you are still following the keto diet because of the variety, richness in flavor and more!

Let's begin.

Table of Contents

Introduction _____ 2

Keto Breakfast Recipes _____ 7

   Keto Cloud Bread _____ 7

   Tasty Yogurt _____ 9

   Avocado Eggs _____ 11

   Keto Brunch _____ 13

   Low Carb Pancakes _____ 15

   Breakfast Burrito _____ 17

   Keto Breakfast Potatoes _____ 19

   Keto Avocado Breakfast Bowl _____ 21

   Steak and Eggs _____ 23

   Keto Bagels _____ 25

   Keto Breakfast Bowl _____ 27

   Chorizo and Eggs _____ 29

Keto Lunch Recipes _____ 31

   Slow Cooker Salsa Verde Chicken _____ 31

   Snow Pea Leaves Stir-Fry _____ 33

   Broccoli Salad with Feta Cheese _____ 35

   Keto Ham & Cheese Pockets _____ 37

   Keto Broccoli Casserole _____ 39

   Avocado Lime Salmon _____ 41

   Broccoli Cheese Soup _____ 43

Keto Pizza — 45

Easy Baked Cauliflower — 48

Brussels Sprouts with Bacon — 50

Keto Dinner Recipes — 52

Slow Cooker Pulled Pork — 52

Fried Chicken with Broccoli — 54

Bunless Burger — 56

Cheese Meatballs — 58

Maple Butter Pork Tenderloin — 60

Baked Chicken Thighs — 62

Caprese Chicken — 64

Keto Desserts — 66

Keto Brownies — 66

Keto Chocolate Mousse — 69

Chocolate Nutella Truffles — 70

Keto No Bake Cookies — 72

Lemon Mousse — 74

Chocolate Coconut Haystack — 76

Keto Peanut Butter Mousse — 78

Keto Chocolate Cake — 80

Keto Crème Brulee — 82

Keto Chocolate Cookies — 85

Dairy-Free Keto Ice Cream — 87

Chocolate Peanut Clusters 89

Keto Snacks, Side Dishes and Appetizers 90

Cheesy Cauliflower Tots 90

Keto Candied Pecans 93

Butter Pecan Bites 95

Parmesan Zucchini Sticks 97

Yogurt Jello Bites 99

Keto Cookie Bars 101

Keto Cookies 103

Jalapeno Poppers Fat Bombs 105

Cauliflower Mash 107

Peanut Butter Cookies 109

Low Carb Chicken Nuggets 111

Keto Eggs 113

Spicy Roasted Nuts 115

Conclusion 117

Keto Breakfast Recipes

Keto Cloud Bread

Yields: 10 pieces

Prep time: 10 minutes

Cook time: 30 minutes

Total time: 40 minutes

Ingredients

¼ teaspoon of salt

¼ teaspoon cream of tartar

3 tablespoons of cream cheese, softened

3 eggs, room temperature

Directions

Preheat your oven to 300 degrees F and prepare 2 baking sheets by lining with parchment paper.

Carefully separate the egg yolks from the egg whites then place them in separate bowls.

Add the cream cheese to the bowl with the egg yolks then use a hand mixer to mix until well combined.

Add the cream of tartar and salt to the other bowl with the egg whites then mix together at high speed using a hand mixer until stiff peaks form.

Use a spoon or spatula to add the yolk mixture to the egg white mix, and fold in carefully until there are no white streaks.

Spoon the mixture onto the lined baking sheet to about ½-3/4 inches tall leaving about 5 inches space between each.

Place in the oven in the middle rack and bake until the tops are lightly golden brown; this should take about 30 minutes.

Allow to cool as they will be too crumbly straight from the oven. Enjoy.

Nutritional information per serving: Calories 35, Proteins 2.2g, Carbs 0.4g and Fats 2.8g

Tasty Yogurt

Yields: 4 Servings

Prep Time: 5 minutes

Cook Time: 10 minutes

Total Time: 15 minutes

Ingredients

400 ml of coconut cream

2 whole probiotic pills powdered form

1 teaspoon of Guar Gum

Directions

Add coconut cream to your saucepan then add the guar gum and start to heat the cream slowly until it starts to boil.

Once the cream is boiling, keep simmering for 7 minutes.

Remove from heat then allow it to cool to about 42 degrees C (108 degrees F).

Once cooled, transfer to a glass jar then add in the probiotic tablet powder. Stir using a sterilized spoon then cover with a piece of cheesecloth, secure with a rubber band around the top and let this sit for 48 hours in a warm place. You can also make it easier by pouring into a thermos to maintain the temp at/or around 42 degrees C for longer.

Nutritional information per serving: Calories 184, Proteins 2g, Carbs 1g and Fats 17g

Avocado Eggs

Yields: 2 Servings

Prep Time: 5 minutes

Cook Time: 14 minutes

Total Time: 19 minutes

Ingredients

1 tablespoon of cheese

1 piece of bacon, cooked and crumbled

2 eggs

1 medium avocado

Pinch of salt

Directions

Preheat your oven to 425 degrees F.

Cut your avocado in half then remove the pit.

Scoop out some of the avocado using a spoon so that the space inside is a little bigger then place in a muffin pan to stabilize the avocado while cooking.

Crack your egg into the avocado then sprinkle with a bit of cheese, a pinch of salt and finally, top with cooked bacon.

Cook for 14 to 16 minutes and serve warm.

Nutritional information per serving: Calories 125, Proteins 8g, Carbs 0g and Fats 9g

Keto Brunch

Yields: 4 servings

Prep Time: 10 minutes

Cook Time: 20 minutes

Total Time: 30 minutes

Ingredients

12 slices of pastured, sugar free bacon

24 asparagus spears

4 large eggs

Directions

Pre-heat your oven to 400F.

Trim the asparagus around an inch from the bottoms. Wrap them in pairs with one slice of bacon. With the asparagus held firmly and close together with one hand, wind the bacon from the bottom to the top of the spear. As you wind the bacon, gently pull it so that it wraps tightly then place on a sheet pan.

Repeat with the rest of the asparagus to have 12 pairs wrapped with bacon.

Place in the oven and set your timer for 20 minutes.

Meanwhile, add water to a small pot and bring to a rapid boil then gently add in the eggs then set another timer for 6 minutes.

Add ice water to a bowl. Once the 6 minutes are up, transfer the eggs quickly to the ice bath using tongs or a slotted spoon. Let the eggs sit for 2 minutes before you peel the tops off.

Crack the top of the egg gently on a hard surface then peel off the shell to expose the tip of the egg.

Serve the asparagus on a cutting board or tray once they are done baking. Hold your eggs up in an egg holder. If you don't have an egg holder just use espresso cups.

Scoop out the tops of the soft boiled eggs using a small spoon to reveal a perfectly runny yolk.

Dip the bacon wrapped asparagus spears into the eggs and enjoy.

Nutritional information per serving: Calories 426, Proteins 17g, Carbs 3g and Fats 38g

Low Carb Pancakes

Yields: about 5-6 small pancakes

Prep time: 2 minutes

Cook time: 15 minutes

Total time: 17 minutes

Ingredients

1 teaspoon of vanilla extract

2 tablespoons of coconut flour

2 eggs

2 oz. of Cream Cheese

Dash of salt

Optional:

Dash of cinnamon

Directions

Add all ingredients to your blender and blend until all ingredients are completely blended together.

Cook the pancakes until you finish the pancake batter.

Keto in Five

Nutritional information per serving: Calories 207, Proteins 9.5g, Carbs 4.2g and Fats 15.3g

Breakfast Burrito

Yields: 1 burrito

Prep Time: 5 minutes

Cook Time: 2 minutes

Total Time: 7 minutes

Ingredients

2 tablespoons of full-fat cream

2 medium eggs

1 tablespoon of butter

Salt/pepper to taste

Choice of herbs or spices

Directions

Whisk the cream, eggs, chosen spices and herbs in a small bowl.

Add butter to your frying pan, and let it melt. Once melted, pour in the egg mixture. Swirl the pan until the mixture is thin and evenly spread. Cover with a lid then allow the burrito to cook for 2 minutes.

Using a clean spatula, gently lift the burrito and transfer to a plate. Add your desired Keto friendly fillings then roll it up and enjoy.

Nutritional information per serving: Calories 331, Proteins 11g, Carbs 1g and Fats 30g

Keto Breakfast Potatoes

Yields: 4 servings

Prep time: 5 minutes

Cook time: 15 minutes

Total time: 20 minute

Ingredients

3 slices of bacon

¼ onion, diced

Salt and pepper to taste

1 tablespoon of olive oil

1 large turnip, peeled and diced

Directions

Add oil to a large skillet then place over medium high heat. Add in the spices and turnips then cook for 5 to 7 minutes making sure that you stir occasionally.

Add in the onion and cook until it starts to soften; takes around 3 minutes. Chop up the bacon into small pieces then add in the skillet. Keep cooking until the bacon is crispy; this should take 5 to 7 more minutes.

Serve and enjoy.

Nutritional information per serving: Calories 88, Proteins 3g, Carbs 4g and Fats 6g

Keto Avocado Breakfast Bowl

Yields: 2 Avocado Bowls

Prep Time: 5 minutes

Cook Time: 15 minutes

Total Time: 20 minutes

Ingredients

3 rashers of bacon, cut into small pieces

3 large free range eggs

1 tablespoon of salted butter

1 avocado, halved and the stone removed

Pinch of salt and black pepper

Directions

Scoop out most of the avocado flesh to leave about ½ inch all-round the avocado.

Heat a large saucepan over low heat then add in the butter. Crack the eggs into a bowl and beat them while the butter is melting then season the eggs with a pinch of pepper and salt.

Add in the bacon to one side of the saucepan then allow them to cook for a few minutes. Add the eggs to the other side of the saucepan and stir regularly to scramble. The bacon and the eggs should all be done 5 minutes after adding the eggs to the pan. If your eggs are done before the bacon is, remove the eggs and place them in a bowl

Add the scrambled eggs and bacon pieces to a bowl and mix together then spoon the mixture into the avocado bowls.

Nutritional information per serving: Calories 500, Proteins 25g, Carbs 3g and Fats 40g

Steak and Eggs

Yields: 1 serving

Prep time: 10 minutes

Cook time: 5 minutes

Total time: 15 minutes

Ingredients

¼ avocado

4 oz. of sirloin

3 eggs

1 tablespoon of butter

Salt and pepper

Directions

Add butter to your pan then melt.

Fry 2-3 eggs in the pan until the yolk is to your desired doneness and the whites are set. Season with pepper and salt

Cook the sirloin (or your preferred cut of steak) in another pan to your desired doneness. Slice the cooked steak into bite-sized strips then season with pepper and salt

Slice up the avocado and serve together with the steak and eggs.

Nutritional information per serving: Calories 510, Proteins 44g, Carbs 3g and Fats 36g

Keto Bagels

Yields: 6 bagels

Prep time: 5 minutes

Cook time: 12 minutes

Total time: 17 minutes

Ingredients

¾ cup of almond flour

1 teaspoon of baking powder

1 oz. of cream cheese

1 1/2 cups of shredded mozzarella cheese

1 large egg

Directions

Preheat your oven to 400 degrees F then prepare your baking sheet by lining with parchment paper.

Add the cream cheese and mozzarella to a microwave safe bowl and microwave for 30 seconds on high. Using a fork, stir to combine then place back in the microwave until fully melted for another 30 seconds.

Add in the baking powder, egg and almond flour then stir to combine using the fork. Use a spatula or your hands to mix until the mixture is uniform in consistency and texture.

Portion the dough into 6 equal balls. Using your hands, roll out each ball into a thin log then form a circle on the parchment. Repeat with the rest of the dough.

To help the seasoning stick better, brush the top of each bagel lightly with some water. Sprinkle the bagels with Everything bagel seasoning then lightly press down with your fingers.

Bake for 12 to 14 minutes

Nutritional information per serving: Calories: 191, Carbs: 4g, Protein: 10g, Fat: 15g

Keto Breakfast Bowl

Yields: 1 serving

Prep time: 10 minutes

Cook time: 0 minutes

Total time: 10 minutes

Ingredients

For the overnight Matcha chia bowl

1-2 teaspoons Matcha to taste (this recipe uses 2 teaspoons)

2 tablespoons of chia seeds

1 cup of almond or coconut milk

Pinch of pink Himalayan salt

Vanilla stevia drops to taste

Directions

Mix together the chia seeds with the sweetener, matcha, your chosen milk and salt then cover and refrigerate overnight. For the milk, this recipe mixed 1-2 tablespoons of full fat coconut milk with 1 cup of water.

You can add as much liquid as you want to achieve your desired consistency. Sweeten then serve with the topping of your choice.

Serving suggestions (optional)

Fresh strawberries

Lightly toasted Almonds

Lightly toasted shredded coconut

Nutritional information per serving: Calories 151, Proteins 5g, Carbs 1.5g and Fats 10g

Chorizo and Eggs

Yields: 2 servings

Prep time: 10 minutes

Cook time: 10 minutes

Total time: 20 minutes

Ingredients

4 eggs

2 (3-ounce) chorizo sausages

1/2 small yellow onion (chopped)

1 teaspoon olive oil

Salt and pepper to taste

Directions

Slice the sausage casings open then spoon the meat into a bowl. Set aside.

In a large skillet, heat the oil over medium high heat. Add in the onions and cook until browned for 3 to 4 minutes then stir in the sausage. Cook until the sausage is cooked through then spread it in the skillet evenly.

Crack in the eggs then season with pepper and salt. Using a wooden spoon, break up the yolks a little bit, stirring the eggs in the sausage.

Cook until the yolks are done to your liking and the egg white are firm. Serve hot.

Nutritional information per serving: Calories 555, Proteins 33g, Carbs 3.5g and Fats 45g

Keto Lunch Recipes

Slow Cooker Salsa Verde Chicken

Yields: 12 servings

Prep Time: 1 minute

Cook Time: 6-7 hours

Total Time: 6 hours 1 minute

Ingredients

1 cup of store-bought salsa verde

3 lb. boneless, skinless chicken breasts or thighs

1 teaspoon of sea salt

Directions

Evenly sprinkle the chicken with sea salt then place in your slow cooker. Add in the salsa verde and mix together with the chicken. Cook on LOW for 6-7 hours or on HIGH for 3-4 hours.

Transfer the chicken to a bowl or cutting board once it's done cooking and shred using 2 forks.

Place the chicken back in the slow cooker and stir in the salsa. Keep the chicken on low until you are ready to eat.

Nutritional information per serving: Calories 138, Proteins 24g, Carbs 1g, Fats 3g

Snow Pea Leaves Stir-Fry

Yields: 2 servings

Prep time: 10 Minutes

Cook time: 4 Minutes

Total time: 14 Minutes

Ingredients

3 tablespoons of avocado oil

3-4 garlic cloves, finely chopped

1 lb. snow pea leaves

Salt to taste

Directions

Wash or rinse the snow pea leaves in water at room temperature then drain using a salad spinner or simply set aside to drain well. Meanwhile, prepare the garlic.

Preheat a wok or a large sauté skillet over medium high heat then add the avocado oil once hot. Reduce heat to medium then add the garlic. Season with a pinch of salt then sauté for about 5-8 seconds until fragrant.

Add in the snow pea leaves then increase the heat to medium high. Using chopsticks or tongs to gently toss the leaves.

For the entire batch to cook evenly, toss often (takes a total of about 3-4 minutes). The stem parts should still be tender and crisp yet the leafy part should turn a deeper vibrant green color. Season with salt to taste.

Remove from heat then transfer to a large serving plate. Serve the garlic over the greens. You may leave behind any juices in the skillet if you wish or add them to your meal.

Serve immediately at room temp or chilled slightly with some steak or chicken

Nutritional information per serving: Calories 239, Proteins 7g, Carbs 3g and Fats 22g

Broccoli Salad with Feta Cheese

Yields: 4 servings

Prep Time: 15 minutes

Cook time: 5 minutes

Total Time: 20 minutes

Ingredients

1 ½ teaspoons of lime juice

1 tablespoon of olive oil

1 head of broccoli - generally 3 stalks for about 3 cups of ribbons yield

¼ cup of crumbled feta cheese

Salt and pepper to taste

Directions

To make the broccoli ribbons, cut the florets from the broccoli stalk so that you remain with a log shaped stalk. Set the florets aside for another use.

Cut the logs in halves then cut the halves in half.

Lay the cut logs smooth side up on a cutting board then make ribbons using a vegetable peeler making sure you stop before getting to the tough outer layer.

Place the ribbons in a serving bowl then toss with lime juice and olive oil; season with pepper and salt.

If using the cheese, top with feta cheese.

Nutritional information per serving: Calories 79, Proteins 3g, Carbs 5g and Fats 5g

Keto Ham & Cheese Pockets

Yields: 2 servings

Prep time: 10 minutes

Cook time: 20 minutes

Total time: 30 minutes

Ingredients

3 oz. slices provolone cheese

3 oz. of quality ham

4 tablespoons of flax meal

1 heaped tablespoon of cream cheese

¾ cup of shredded mozzarella

Directions

Prepare the dough by melting the cream cheese and shredded mozzarella in the microwave for 1 minute. Check halfway through and mix then return back to the microwave.

Add in the flax meal and stir until the dough is well combined.

Roll out the dough between 2 sheets of parchment. Add the cheese slices and ham and then like an envelope, fold over and seal the dough. Poke holes on the dough to release steam during baking.

Bake for 15-20 minutes at 400 degrees until firm to the touch and golden brown. Remove from the oven once done and allow it to cool down for a few minutes then cut in half and enjoy while hot.

You can also allow it to cool down completely then refrigerate for up to 3 days.

Nutritional information per serving: Calories 426, Proteins 31.7g, Carbs 4.2g and Fats 31g

Keto Broccoli Casserole

Yields: 4 servings

Prep time: 5 minutes

Active time: 20 minutes

Total time: 25 minutes

Ingredients

1 cup of grated cheese

½ cup of sour cream

½ cup of cream

1 head of broccoli

Directions

Preheat your oven to 350 degrees F and get an oven proof dish.

Cut the broccoli into bite sized pieces then put them into the oven proof dish. Add in the sour cream and cream then stir to coat the broccoli well with both creams.

Add in a third of the cheese and mix until combined well then top with the remaining cheese.

Bake in the oven until golden and crisp for 15 to 20 minutes.

Nutritional information per serving: Calories 218, Proteins 10.1g, Carbs 0g and Fats 10.8g

Avocado Lime Salmon

Yields: 2 servings

Prep time: 20 minutes

Cook time: 10 minutes

Total time: 30 minutes

Ingredients

100 grams of cauliflower

2 tablespoons of red onion (diced)

½ lime

1 avocado

2 salmon fillets (6 oz.)

Directions

Rice the cauliflower by placing in your food processor and pulsing until it resembles rice. Cook covered for 8 minutes in a lightly oiled pan.

Blend together the diced red onion, the juice of ½ a lime and avocado in a food processor until creamy and smooth.

Add some oil to a skillet and heat then cook the salmon fillet for about 4-5 minutes with the skin side down; season with pepper and salt while cooking. Flip over the salmon and cook for another 4-5 minutes

Serve over a bed of cauliflower rice once the salmon is done cooking and top with a generous dollop of the avocado lime sauce

Nutritional information per serving: Calories 420, Proteins 37g, Carbs 5g and Fats 27g

Broccoli Cheese Soup

Yields: 3 servings (1 cup each)

Cook Time: 20 minutes

Total Time: 20 minutes

Ingredients

3 cups of cheddar cheese (pre-shredded)

1 cup of heavy cream

3 ½ cups of chicken broth (or bone broth, or vegetable broth)

4 cloves of garlic (minced)

4 cups of broccoli (cut into florets)

Directions

Sauté the garlic in a large pot over medium heat until fragrant for 1 minute.

Add in the chopped broccoli, heavy cream and chicken broth then increase heat and bring to a boil. Lower the heat and simmer until the broccoli is tender for 10-20 minutes.

Remove about 1/3 of the broccoli pieces using a slotted spoon and set aside (this is completely optional if you would like your soup to have some pieces at the end. You can leave them in if you want all the soup pureed).

Puree the remaining broccoli using an immersion blender

Reduce the heat to low then add in the shredded cheddar cheese half a cup at a time stirring constantly and keep stirring until melted. To make the soup smooth, puree again.

Remove from heat and add in the reserved broccoli florets.

Nutritional information per serving: Calories 291, Proteins 13g, Carbs 4g and Fats 25g

Keto Pizza

Yields: 4-6 servings

Prep Time: 10 minutes

Cook Time: 15 minutes

Total Time: 25 minutes

Ingredients

For the keto pizza fathead crust

1 egg beaten

2 oz. of full-fat cream cheese, room temp

¾ cup of blanched almond flour

1 ½ cups of part skim mozzarella, shredded

Optional: 1 teaspoon of oregano

Directions

Begin by preparing all the ingredients. Crack the egg in a small bowl, sift the almond flour and shred the mozzarella cheese.

Preheat your oven to 425 degrees F.

Add the cream cheese, almond flour and the shredded low moisture mozzarella cheese to a microwave safe bowl. Stir until combined well

Place the cheese mixture in the microwave and microwave for about 90-120 seconds, stirring halfway through.

Remove the melted mixture from the microwave and stir in the beaten egg using wooden spoon or spatula.

Oil your hands then knead the dough into a ball. Roll the dough to 1/4" or 1/3" thickness between 2 sheets of parchment paper. Poke holes through the pizza crust using a fork.

Bake until the crust looks golden for 6-8 minutes.

Allow the pizza crust to cool on a cooling rack while still on the baking sheet then add your desired toppings. Check the toppings suggestions below. This recipe used pepperoni slices, mozzarella cheese and marinara sauce

Place the pizza back in the oven and bake until the cheese on top melts beautifully for a few more minutes.

Slice the pizza into 4 or 6 pieces and enjoy.

Toppings suggestions

Vegetables: mushrooms, ¼ chopped red pepper

Sauce: olive oil, pesto, 3 tablespoons of sugar-free tomato sauce

Meats: chose from 12 slices of pepperoni, bacon, turkey, ham, beef, chicken

Cheese: ¼ cup mozzarella cheese, Gouda, feta, blue, parmesan, and fresh mozzarella cheeses etc.

Oregano to garnish

Nutritional information per serving: Calories 289, Proteins 16g, Carbs 4g and Fats 22g

Easy Baked Cauliflower

Yields: 6 servings

Prep time: 5 minutes

Cook time: 25 minutes

Total time: 30 minutes

Ingredients

1 large cauliflower

½ cup of extra virgin olive oil

1 teaspoon of sea salt

1 teaspoon of "Herbes De Provence"

4 garlic cloves, peeled

Directions

Preheat your oven to 400 degrees F.

Mix the oil, herbs, salt and garlic in a small food processor until smooth and creamy.

Wash the cauliflower thoroughly from the hardcore to the bottom leaves then slice into thick slices.

Place the cauliflower pieces and slices on a large cookie sheet – they may crumble and break a bit.

Using a fork or a pastry brush, brush the cauliflower with the garlic and oil cream.

Bake until the bottom part is brown for about 25 minutes then flip and bake until the other side is also browned for 15 more minutes.

Serve warm as a side dish to chicken or whatever meat you prefer.

Nutritional information per serving: Calories 197, Proteins 2.8g, Carbs 4.5g and Fats 19g

Brussels Sprouts with Bacon

Yields: 4 servings

Prep time: 5 minutes

Cook time: 30 minutes

Total time: 35 minutes

Ingredients

8 strips of bacon

2 tablespoons of olive oil

1 lb. of Brussels sprouts

Salt and pepper

Directions

Preheat your oven to 375 degrees F.

Cut off the ends of each Brussels sprout then cut each in half. If they are very big you can cut them even into quarters.

Toss the chopped Brussels in a deep bowl with olive oil, pepper, salt and any other spices you like such as cumin and red pepper.

Prepare your baking sheet by greasing then place the Brussels on top ensuring you leave a bit of space between them.

Place in the oven and bake for about 30 minutes stopping halfway through to shake the baking sheet so that the Brussels flip or rotate a little.

Fry as much bacon as you like while the Brussels sprouts are baking. This recipe uses 2 pieces of bacon per serving.

Chop the bacon up into small pieces once it is cooked to your liking – the pieces should be roughly half an inch (bite sized).

The Brussels sprouts are ready when they are blackened and shriveled a bit. Remove from oven and toss them in the bowl with the bits of bacon.

Serve and sprinkle with a bit of salt.

Nutritional information per serving: Calories 278, Proteins 15g, Carbs 4g and Fats 21g

Keto Dinner Recipes

Slow Cooker Pulled Pork

Yields: 14 servings

Prep Time: 5 minutes

Ingredients

7 lbs. of pork shoulder roast

2 cups of sugar-free barbecue sauce

3 cans of natural stevia-sweetened root beer

2 teaspoons of paprika

1 teaspoon each of garlic powder and onion powder

Directions

Remove the twine from the pork butt then put into your slow cooker.

Sprinkle with onion powder, garlic powder and paprika. Add the root beer along the side of the pork. Cover the slow cooker with a lid and cook for 9 hours on low.

Drain the pork juices from the cooker then return the meat back and shred using a fork

Add the barbecue then cover and cook for 1 more hour on low.

Serve with veggies.

Nutritional Information Per Serving: Calories 405, Proteins 31.8g, Carbs 2.4g and Fats 29.2g

Fried Chicken with Broccoli

Yields: 2 servings

Prep time: 5 minutes

Cook time: 15 minutes

Total time: 20 minutes

Ingredients

10 ounces of boneless chicken thighs

3½ ounces of butter

9 ounces of broccoli

Salt and pepper

Optional: ½ cup of mayonnaise, for serving

Directions

Rinse the broccoli and trim then cut into smaller pieces including the stem.

Add a generous dollop of butter to a frying pan that can fit both the broccoli and the chicken then heat it up.

Season the chicken then fry over medium heat in the pan with butter for around 5 minutes per side, until cooked through and golden brown.

Add more butter to the pan then place in the broccoli. Fry for a couple more minutes and season

Serve with the remaining butter

Nutritional information per serving: Calories 733, Proteins 29g, Carbs 5g and Fats 66g

Bunless Burger

Yields: 3 Servings

Prep Time: 5 minutes

Cook Time: 10 minutes

Total Time: 15 minutes

Ingredients

1 tablespoon of McCormicks Montreal Steak Seasoning

1 tablespoon of Worcestershire sauce

1 pound of ground beef

Salt and pepper

Optional

4 ounces of sliced onion

2 tablespoons of bacon drippings or olive oil

Directions

Preheat your grill and clean the grate.

Break the ground beef up then distribute the Worcestershire sauce evenly and steak seasoning; add the olive oil here if using.

To distribute the seasoning, mix gently with your hands then form into 3 balls. Gently pat/press into patties or just use a burger press. To prevent the burger from puffing up in the middle, make a slight depression in the center.

Oil the grate then season both sides of the burger with a light sprinkling of pepper and salt. Grill to your preferred level of doneness.

Optional: To make the caramelized onions, slice the onions first. Place your pan over medium low heat then add in 1 tablespoon of oil. Once hot, add in the onions and sauté until softened. Add in half a teaspoon of erythritol and cook until they start to caramelize or brown; this can take up to 10 minutes

Nutritional information per serving: Calories: 479, Carbohydrates: 2g, Protein: 26g and Fat: 40g

Notes

Nutritional info for one burger with 1/3 of the Caramelized Onions: Calories: 531, Protein: 26 g, Carbohydrates 5g, Fat: 45g, Fiber: 1g, NET CARBS: 4g.

Cheese Meatballs

Yields: 3 Servings

Prep Time: 10 minutes

Cook Time: 10 minutes

Total Time: 20 minutes

Ingredients

1 teaspoon of garlic powder

3 tablespoons of parmesan cheese

100 g of cheese - mozzarella works best

500g of beef mince (ground beef)

½ teaspoon each of salt and pepper

Directions

Cut the cheese into cubes of 1cm by 1 cm.

Mix the ground beef with the dry ingredients then wrap the cheese cubes in mince – you should get about 9 balls from 500g of mince.

Fry the meatballs in the pan and serve the meatballs with sautéed vegetables.

Nutritional information per serving: Calories 444, Proteins 46g, Carbs 2g and Fats 28g

Maple Butter Pork Tenderloin

Yields: 8 Servings

Prep Time: 5 minutes

Cook Time: 25 minutes

Total Time: 30 minutes

Ingredients

2-3 pounds Pork Tenderloin trimmed of silver skin

¼ cup of sugar free maple syrup

½ yellow onion, thinly sliced

8 tablespoons of butter

Salt and Pepper

Directions

Preheat your oven to 350 degrees F.

Place a large oven safe skillet over medium high heat then add the butter once hot and stir until melted.

Add in the maple syrup and stir then simmer for about 1 minute.

Season the pork tenderloin with pepper and salt on all sides then add to the skillet carefully.

Without moving or turning it in the pan, cook the pork for 5 minutes then flip and cook the other side for another 5 minutes.

Arrange the sliced onions carefully in the skillet around the pork then transfer the pork to the oven and bake for about 10 minutes until it reaches a minimum internal temp of 45 degrees F.

Transfer the pork tenderloins to a serving tray to rest before you slice it up.

Meanwhile, place back the skillet over medium high heat. Allow the onions, syrup and butter to simmer while you stir frequently until the sauce has reduced by about half and the onions are translucent and soft.

Slice the pork and serve topped with the reduced sauce and onions from the skillet with some vegetables. Enjoy

Nutritional information per serving: Calories 240, Proteins 23g, Carbs 0g and Fats 15g

Baked Chicken Thighs

Yield: 9 servings

Prep Time: 15 minutes

Cook Time: 30 minutes

Total Time: 45 minutes

Ingredients

2 teaspoons of oregano, dried

2–3 large garlic cloves, grated

3 pounds chicken thighs bone in and skin on

1 teaspoon of salt

Ground black pepper, to taste

For garnish: Parsley or dill, finely chopped

Directions

Add the oregano, garlic, chicken thighs, pepper and salt to an 8 x 8 square baking dish. Toss to coat using your hands then let this stand for 10 minutes.

Preheat the oven to 450 degrees F.

Toss the chicken again ensuring you spread the spices and garlic evenly. Arrange the chicken, skin side up in a single layer, ensuring you tuck the skin underneath – you want to keep it tight.

Bake uncovered for 30-40 minutes until lots of juices accumulate in the dish, the skin starts to brown and the thermometer reads at least 165 degrees F.

Pour juices over the chicken thighs using a baster/syringe then for a crispy skin, broil to your likeness.

Remove from the oven then cover and let it stand for 5 minutes for the juices to settle.

Serve warm without the skin for a healthier version with cauliflower risotto, quinoa or brown rice and a salad.

Nutritional information per serving: Calories 377, Proteins 28.2g, Carbs 0.4g and Fats 28.2g

Caprese Chicken

Yields: 4 servings

Prep Time: 5 minutes

Cook Time: 35 minutes

Total Time: 40 minutes

Ingredients

1 medium tomato sliced into 5 or 6 slices

6 ounces of fresh mozzarella sliced into

5 boneless skinless chicken thighs

¼ cup of fresh basil chopped

2 tablespoons of avocado oil

Directions

Preheat the oven to 375 degrees F.

Heat the oil until simmering in a large skillet over medium heat.

Sprinkle the chicken thighs with pepper and salt then add to the pan in a single layer. Sear for about 2-3 minutes until golden brown then flip and sear the other side for 2-3 more minutes.

Add the chicken to a medium casserole dish or glass baking pan in a single layer. Top each piece with a slice of fresh mozzarella and a slice of tomato.

Bake until the chicken is cooked through and the cheese is melted and bubbling for 25 to 28 minutes. Broil to brown the top of the cheese for 2-3 minutes.

Sprinkle with fresh basil before serving.

Nutritional information per serving: Calories 315, Proteins 35.7g, Carbs 1.63 and Fats 18.7g

Keto Desserts

Keto Brownies

Yields: 16 servings

Prep time: 15 minutes

Cook time: 20 minutes

Total time: 35 minutes

Ingredients

70 g almond flour

2 eggs at room temperature

80 g of cocoa powder

140-200 g xylitol powdered erythritol

130 g of unsalted grass-fed butter

Optional garnish

Flakey sea salt (highly recommended)

Directions

Place the rack in the lower third of your oven then preheat to 350 degrees F.

Prepare an 8x8-inch baking pan by lining the sides and bottom with parchment paper; set aside.

Into a medium heat proof bowl, add the cocoa powder, sweetener and butter then melt over a water bath stirring constantly or in the microwave in small increments. Heat until most of the sweetener is melted and the mixture is incorporated well.

*Note: erythritol will not dissolve much at this point unlike xylitol.

Remove the mixture from heat and allow it to cool slightly.

Crack in the eggs one at a time, whisking well after each addition until incorporated completely. The texture of the resulting mixture should appear smooth with all the sweetener dissolved. You may want to add an extra egg if using erythritol and the batter becomes too thick. Ensure you don't over whisk otherwise you may end up with cakey rather than fudgy brownies

Add in the almond flour and whisk vigorously for about a minute until well mixed.

Bake until the center is set and a toothpick comes out moist when inserted in the center; this takes about 15-25 minutes (about 17 with erythritol and 23 with xylitol) but it really varies from oven to oven so check on them after 15 minutes the first time round.

Sprinkle with the flakey sea salt if desired then place the brownies on a rack to cool completely. Using the edges of the parchment paper, lift the brownies then cut into desired size

*Tip: Place the brownies in the freezer for 10 minutes before cutting to get extra clean edges

SERVING SUGGESTIONS

Unsweetened macadamia milk - nice 'n cold!

Nutritional information per serving: Calories 102, Proteins 2g, Carbs 1g and Fats 9g

Keto Chocolate Mousse

Yields: 4 servings

Prep time: 10 minutes

Cook time: 0 minutes

Total time: 10 minutes

Ingredients

¼ teaspoon of kosher salt

1 teaspoon of vanilla extract

¼ cup of powdered sweetener

¼ cup of unsweetened cocoa powder, sifted

1 cup of heavy whipping cream

Directions

Whisk the heavy cream until stiff peaks form.

Add in the vanilla, sweetener, cocoa powder and salt the whisk until just combined

Nutritional information per serving: Calories 218, Proteins 2g, Carbs 3g and Fats 23g

Chocolate Nutella Truffles

Servings: 16 truffles

Prep Time: 20 minutes

Cook Time: 5 minutes

Total Time: 25 minutes

Ingredients

1/3 cup of powdered erythritol

½ cup of sugar-free dark chocolate chips

½ cup of hazelnuts, chopped very finely

½ cup of Sugar-free "Nutella" spread (or any chocolate hazelnut spread of your choice or regular Nutella if not sugar-free,)*

1/3 cup of coconut oil

Optional: ½ teaspoon of vanilla extract

Directions

In a medium saucepan, combine all ingredients apart from the chopped hazelnuts. Melt until smooth over low heat stirring constantly.

Refrigerate until partially set for 60-90 minutes. Stir then refrigerate for another 1-2 hours until firm.

Spoon round chunks of the batter using a small cookie scoop then form into 2.5-3cm balls. Ensure your hands are cold and that you only use your fingertips to avoid melting.

Roll each ball and press into chopped hazelnuts to coat all over.

Keep refrigerated until ready to serve to keep the truffles firm.

Nutritional information per serving: Calories 78, Proteins 1.5g, Carbs 1.8g and Fats 7.5g

Keto No Bake Cookies

Yields: 20 cookies

Prep Time: 5 minutes

Cook Time: 1 minute

Total Time: 30 minutes

Ingredients

2 tablespoons of butter, melted

2 cups of unsweetened coconut flakes

2 tablespoons of unsweetened cocoa powder

2 teaspoons of vanilla extract

1 1/3 cups of creamy peanut butter

Optional: 1 teaspoon of erythritol

Directions

Prepare a large baking sheet by lining with a non-stick silicone mat or parchment paper.

Combine the cocoa powder, coconut flakes, melted butter, vanilla extract and peanut butter in a large mixing bowl. Stir until well combined. (Feel free to add 1-2 teaspoons of your desired sugar alternative if you like your cookies a little sweeter. The recipe used swerve)

Spoon the batter onto the earlier prepared baking sheet then gently shape each scoop into a 3" cookie using the back of a spoon.

Place the cookies in the freezer to set for 30 minutes.

Store in the freezer in an airtight container

Nutritional information per serving: Calories 153, Proteins 4g, Carbs 4g and Fats 13g

Lemon Mousse

Yields: 2 servings

Prep time: 5 minutes

Cook time: 0 minutes

Total time: 5 minutes

Ingredients

1 cup of cream

2 tablespoons of stevia

1 lemon

½ cup of mascarpone cheese

Directions

Whisk the mascarpone in a bowl until smooth.

Grate the zest from your lemon over the mascarpone then slice in half and squeeze the juice as well. Add in the stevia and whisk until smooth

Whisk the cream until smooth in a separate bowl then pour into the lemon mixture. Taste to know whether you require any extra sweetener then transfer to a serving bowl

To thicken, refrigerate for a few hours. Enjoy.

Nutritional information per serving: Calories, Protein 2g, Carbs 3.5g and Fats 30g

Chocolate Coconut Haystack

Yields: 20 cookies

Prep Time: 20 minutes

Refrigeration time: 1 hour

Total Time: 20 minutes

Ingredients

1 1/3 cups of stevia chocolate chips or regular chocolate chips

2 cups of shredded coconut

Directions

In a double boiler, melt the chocolate until smooth then turn off heat. Ensure you don't overheat the chips.

Place the shredded coconut in a bowl then pour in the melted chocolate, and mix.

Prepare your cookie sheet by lining with parchment paper then form the mixture into a stack on the lined cookie sheet. The mixture will not hold together when wet; it will feel loose.

Refrigerate until hardened for about 1-2 hours.

Nutritional information per serving: Calories 93, Proteins 1.3g, Carbs 3.7g and Fats 8.9g

Keto Peanut Butter Mousse

Yields: 4 servings

Prep Time: 5 minutes

Cook time: 0 minutes

Total Time: 5 minutes

Ingredients

½ teaspoon of vanilla extract

¼ cup of powdered Swerve Sweetener

¼ cup of natural peanut butter (no sugar added)

4 ounces of cream cheese (softened)

½ cup of heavy whipping cream (more if needed to thin the mixture)

Directions

Whip ½ cup of the cream in a medium bowl until it has stiff peaks. Set aside.

Beat together the peanut butter and cream cheese in another medium bowl until creamy and smooth. Add in the vanilla, sweetener, pinch of salt and beat until smooth.

Add about 2 tablespoons of heavy cream to your mixture if it's overly thick and beat until combined to lighten it.

Fold in the whipped cream gently until no streaks remain; pipe or spoon into little dessert glasses.

If desired, drizzle with a little low carb chocolate sauce.

Nutritional Information Per Serving: Calories 325, Carbs 3g, Fat 30g, Protein 5g.

Keto Chocolate Cake

Yields: 12 servings

Prep Time: 10 minutes

Cook Time: 30 minutes

Total Time: 40 minutes

Ingredients

1 ½ cups of powdered erythritol

1/2 cup of ground almonds or almond flour

6 eggs

1 1/3 cup melted butter, unsalted

10.5 ounces of unsweetened chocolate

Directions

Preheat your oven to 340 degrees F. (increase the oven temp by 25 degrees F if baking at high altitude).

Melt the chocolate and butter in the microwave then stir and wait until dissolved. Alternatively, you can gently heat in a water bath. Set aside.

Beat the eggs until foamy in a large bowl then add in the sweetener; mix well

Add in the melted butter and chocolate along with almond flour. Using a spatula or spoon, stir until just combined.

Prepare an 8 inch spring form by lining the bottom with parchment paper and greasing the sides with butter. Pour in the batter and bake on the middle shelf until the top of the cake (especially the middle) is firm to the touch; this should take about 30 minutes.

Let the cake to cool in the tin before removing. Dust with cocoa powder once the cake is completely cooled.

Nutritional information per serving: Calories 389, Proteins 8.1g, Carbs 3g and Fats 37.8g

Keto Crème Brulee

Yields: 4 Servings

Prep Time 10 minutes

Cook Time 30 minutes

Total Time 40 minutes

Ingredients

¼ teaspoons of Vanilla bean powder

¼ cup of erythritol

6 large egg yolks

2 cups of Heavy cream

1 tablespoon of Brandy

Optional toppings

Whipped cream

Powdered erythritol

Directions

Preheat your oven to 350 degrees F then position the rack in the middle of the oven.

Add water to a tea kettle and heat until hot but not boiling. Find a pan that is large enough to fit 4 ramekins and is deep enough to fill water halfway up the sides of the ramekins.

Into a medium bowl, add 1 tablespoon of the granulated sweetener and the egg yolks. Beat well to break up the yolks completely.

Add the heavy cream to a small pot then pour in the vanilla powder and the remaining erythritol. If you prefer using the vanilla extract, add it later.

Heat the pot over medium heat until bubbles begin to simmer around the edge of the pot. Use a whisk to stir occasionally. Remove from heat while pouring the egg yolk slowly into the hot mixture in a thin stream, whisking quickly throughout. Add in the brandy and whisk. (If using the vanilla extract instead, add now)

Divide the mixture between 4 ramekins evenly then place the ramekins in the pan. Fill the pan with hot water until halfway up the sides of your ramekins.

Place the pan in the oven carefully and bake until the center of is barely jiggly or for 30 minutes.

Remove from the oven and cool for an hour in the water bath before placing on a rack to cool completely. Cover the crème brulee using plastic wrap then place in the refrigerator for at least 4 hours (preferably overnight).

Sprinkle ½ teaspoon of sweetener over the top before serving. You can add a dollop of whipped cream over the top and serve.

Nutritional information per serving: Calories 502, Proteins 6g, Carbs 4g and Fats 51g

Keto Chocolate Cookies

Yields: 12 cookies

Prep time: 10 minutes

Cook time: 15 minutes

Total time: 25 minutes

Ingredients

¼ teaspoon of salt

1/3 cup of powdered Erythritol

2/3 cup of unsweetened cacao powder

2 large eggs

1 ¼ cups of almond butter or any other nut or seed butter

Optional: 1/4 teaspoon of cayenne pepper and 10-20 drops liquid Stevia extract

Directions

Preheat your oven to 320 degrees F.

Prepare your baking sheet by lining with nonstick silicon baking mat or parchment paper.

Add the almond butter, unsweetened cacao powder, powdered erythritol, eggs and salt to your food processor (you can also use a spatula or your hands to mix the dough). Process until combined well.

Form 12 equal cookie dough balls using your hands then place the balls onto the earlier prepared baking sheet. Press down on each cookie ball using a fork to flatten to about 1cm thick.

Place the baking sheet in the oven and bake until they crisp up or for about 12 minutes. Remove from the oven once done and allow them to cool down before serving.

Store for up to 5 days in an airtight container or freeze for longer storage.

Nutritional information per serving: Calories 195, Proteins 6.8g, Carbs 2.9g and Fats 14.4g

Dairy-Free Keto Ice Cream

Yields: 5 servings

Prep Time: 2 minutes

Churning: 10 minutes

Total Time: 12 minutes

Ingredients

2 tablespoons of vanilla extract

1/8 teaspoon of pure stevia powder to taste

Heaping 1/3 cup of natural almond butter

1 13.7 oz. can of coconut milk full fat

Directions

In a small blender, blend all the ingredients. Taste and adjust the stevia, salt or vanilla if necessary.

Chill the mixture; place the blender container with the ice cream mixture in the freezer an hour prior to churning so that its very cold but not frozen.

Pour the mixture into an ice cream maker and churn until thickened to soft serve consistency for about 10 minutes.

Pour the ice cream into a loaf pan or shallow dish then place in the freezer for 1 hour.

Thaw for 5-10 minutes on the counter, and then to make scooping easier, dip ice cream scoop in water. Enjoy.

Nutritional information per serving: Calories 219, Proteins 4g, Carbs 3g and Fats 19g

Chocolate Peanut Clusters

Yields: 24 servings

Prep Time: 40 minutes

Cook time: 0 minutes

Total Time: 40 minutes

Ingredients

10 ounces of salted peanuts

6 ounces of sugar-free milk chocolate

½ cup of peanut butter

Directions

Place a heatproof bowl in a pan of barely simmering water then add in the chocolate and peanut butter. Stir until smooth and melted.

Add in the peanuts stirring to coat well. Scoop rounded spoonfuls onto a baking sheet lined with waxed paper and chill for about 30 minutes until firm – make the clusters as big or small as you like).

Nutritional information per serving: Calories 132, Proteins 3.92g, Carbs 5g and Fats 11.35g

Keto Snacks, Side Dishes and Appetizers

Cheesy Cauliflower Tots

Yields: 8 servings

Prep Time: 5 minutes

Cook Time: 15 minutes

Total Time: 20 minutes

Ingredients

1 ½ cups of mozzarella cheese

1 large egg

¼ cup of avocado oil; divided

1 ½ pounds of cauliflower (riced, measured after ricing, about 1 head)

¾ teaspoon of sea salt

Optional: 2 cloves of Garlic (minced)

Directions

In a large sauté pan or wok, stir-fry the cauliflower rice in 2 tablespoons of oil over medium high heat until lightly browned and soft without any moisture being left behind in the pan.

Meanwhile, in a large bowl, whisk the egg then mix in the garlic, mozzarella and sea salt.

Once the cauliflower rice is done cooking, transfer to the bowl immediately while still hot then stir it in to make the mixture sticky and melt the cheese.

Scoop balls of the "dough" using a small cookie scoop then form small tarter tot sized patties. Flatten the patties slightly to ensure they are not too thick to cook through well.

Using a paper towel, wipe the pan to get rid of any pieces of the cauliflower rice.

Heat the remaining 2 tablespoons of avocado oil in the pan you just wiped then place over medium heat. Add in the tater tots in a single layer ensuring that they don't touch. Fry until golden on the bottom for about 2 minutes.

Flip and cook until the other side is golden. Transfer the tater tots to a paper towel to drain, and repeat with the rest of the tots (you might need to add more oil in between batches).

Serving size: 6 tater tots

Nutritional information per serving: Calories 142, Proteins 7g, Carbs 3g and Fats 11g

Keto Candied Pecans

Yields: about 6 servings

Prep time: 5 minutes

Cook time: 10 minutes

Total time: 15 minutes

Ingredients

1 teaspoon of vanilla extract

½ cup of monk fruit

¼ cup of butter, unsalted

1 ½ cup of whole pecan halves

Directions

Add butter to a saucepan and melt over medium heat.

Add the monk fruit into the saucepan once the butter is melted and stir constantly until well mixed.

Add in the vanilla extract and stir to combine. Keep cooking the mixture for 7-8 minutes stirring frequently until it begins to thicken.

Turn off heat then add in the pecan halves. Toss to coat all the pecans well then place them on a baking sheet lined with parchment paper in a single layer.

Place the baking sheet in the refrigerator for 1-2 hours for the pecans to harden and cool.

Break any chunks of pecans apart once ready and serve as is.

Store any leftovers in an airtight container.

Nutritional information per serving: Calories 259, Proteins 3.08g, Carbs 1g and Fats 27.7g

Butter Pecan Bites

Yields: 9 servings

Prep time: 10 minutes

Cook time: 0 minutes

Total time: 1 hour 10 minutes

Ingredients

½ teaspoon of sugar-free vanilla extract

1 tablespoon of heavy cream

2 ounces of pecan halves

4 tablespoons of butter, melted

1 tablespoon erythritol

Directions

Melt the butter in your microwave or in a small pot over low heat.

Add in the rest of the ingredients; mix thoroughly

Pour the pecan mass in a suitable silicone mold and chill for at least 1 hour in the fridge.

Pop the pecan bites from the mold and serve with a hot cup of coffee or tea

Store for up to 1 week covered with plastic wrap or in an airtight container

Nutritional information per serving (1 bite): Calories 101, Proteins 4.9g, Carbs 1.1g and Fats 6.4g

Parmesan Zucchini Sticks

Yields: 16 servings

Prep Time: 5 minutes

Cook Time: 20 minutes

Total Time: 25 minutes

Ingredients

½ teaspoon of freshly ground black pepper

¼ teaspoon of salt

½ tablespoon of dried thyme or oregano

1 cup of Parmesan cheese, shredded

8 medium zucchini, cut in half

Directions

Preheat your oven to 350 degrees F. Prepare 2 rimmed baking sheet by lining with parchment paper then arrange the zucchini halves on top.

Mix the black pepper, oregano (or thyme), parmesan cheese and salt in a small bowl.

Top each slice of zucchini with 1-1 ½ tablespoons of cheese herb mixture making sure that you spread the mixture evenly.

Bake for 15 minutes then broil for 4-5 minutes on high or until the cheese is golden and crisp..

Serve cold or warm.

Store any leftover in the refrigerator covered for up to 2-3 days.

Nutritional information per serving: Calories 22, Proteins 2.1g, Carbs 05g and Fats 1.4g

Yogurt Jello Bites

Yields: 6 servings

Prep time: 5 minutes

Cook time: 2 minutes

Cool time: 3 hours

Total time: 7 minutes

Ingredients

0.3 oz. packet Strawberry Sugar Free Jello

16 oz. Greek yogurt

Directions

Mix the ingredients together in a medium bowl then place the bowl in the microwave. Microwave for 1 minute then stir well and microwave in 30 second bursts until the jello crystals have dissolved into the yoghurt completely – stir well during each burst.

Prepare a silicon mold by spraying with some nonstick spray then spoon the mixture into the prepared mold. Use an icing spatula to level off the mold. To remove any air bubbles, tap the mold a few times for at least 3 hours until set.

Place the silicone mold on a board then place in the refrigerator.

Turn out each yoghurt bite carefully and enjoy.

Store any leftovers in the fridge

Nutritional information per serving (3 bites): Calories 47, Proteins 7g, Carbs 3g and Fats 0g

Keto Cookie Bars

Yields: 16 Servings

Prep Time: 10 minutes

Ingredients

1 ¼ cup of raw sesame seeds

¼ teaspoon of grey sea salt

¼ cup of unsweetened apple sauce

¾ cup of coconut butter

Optional

5-10 drops of alcohol-free stevia

½ teaspoon of vanilla extract

½ teaspoon of ground cinnamon

Directions

Preheat your oven to 350 degrees F. Set aside a 16 count silicon baking mold or small muffin silicon molds.

Into a large bowl, add the applesauce, sea salt and coconut butter. If using the optional ingredients, add them in now. Stir until combined fully.

Sprinkle in the sesame seeds then stir to coat.

Press the mixture onto the earlier prepared mold then place in the oven and bake until the tops brown; this should take 10-15 minutes.

Remove from the oven once done then allow the cookies to cool in the molds for 20 minutes. Place in the freezer to firm up for 20 minutes.

Store leftovers at room temperature.

Nutritional information per serving: Calories 120, Proteins 2.4g, Carbs 2.1g and Fats 11g

Keto Cookies

Yields: 10 cookies

Prep time: 10 minutes

Cook time: 15 minutes

Total time: 25 minutes

Ingredients

1 large egg

¼ cup of powdered Erythritol or Swerve

¼ cup of coconut butter - you can make your own

¼ teaspoon of salt

8.8 ounces Almond & Cashew Butter or almond butter

Optional: 1-2 teaspoons of cinnamon or pumpkin spice or vanilla

Directions

Preheat your oven to 320 degrees F.

Mix softened coconut butter with the nut butter then add in the egg, salt and powdered erythritol. Mix until combined well.

Form small cookie dough balls each of about 1 ½ oz. using your hands then place the balls on a baking sheet lined with nonstick silicon baking mat or parchment paper.

Press down on each ball using a fork until about ½ inch thick.

Place the baking sheet in the oven and bake until lightly browned for about 12 minutes.

Be careful not to burn the cookies – nuts burn faster compared to regular flour cookies.

Remove from the oven once done and allow the cookies to cool down. The cookies with harden as they chill.

Store for up to a week in an airtight container or freeze for up to 3 months.

Nutritional information per serving: Calories 204, Proteins 5.1g, Carbs 3.2g and Fats 19.1g

Jalapeno Poppers Fat Bombs

Yields: 6 Servings

Prep Time: 10 minutes

Cook Time: 30 minutes

Total Time: 40 minutes

Ingredients

2 jalapeño peppers halved, seeded, and finely chopped

¼ cup of grated Cheddar cheese or Gruyère cheese

4 slices of no sugar bacon

¼ cup of unsalted butter at room temperature

3.5 ounces of full-fat cream cheese at room temperature

Directions

Preheat your oven to 160 degrees C/ 325 degrees F or gas mark 3.

Prepare a rimmed baking sheet by lining with parchment paper. Ensure you use a rimmed baking sheet so that is contains the bacon fat as it's required for the recipe.

Mash together the butter (or ghee) and cream cheese in a bowl or process until smooth in a food processor.

Lay the bacon slices flat onto the lined baking sheet ensuring that they don't overlap.

Place the baking sheet in the oven and bake until the bacon is crispy for 25 to 30 minutes. The thickness of the bacon determines the exact cooking time.

Remove the bacon from the oven and let it sit to cool. Crumble the bacon into a bowl once cool enough to handle. Set aside.

Add the cheddar or Gruyere cheese, bacon grease and jalapenos to the butter cream cheese mixture. Mix well to combine then refrigerate until set for 30 minutes to 1 hour.

Portion the mixture into 6 equal fat bombs then place them on a plate lined with parchment. Roll the bombs in the crumbled bacon if serving immediately until well coated. If saving them for later, refrigerate in an airtight container without the bacon coating for up to 1 week. Roll them in reheated or freshly cooked bacon crumbs right before serving.

Nutritional information per serving: Calories 208, Proteins 4g, Carbs 1g and Fats 20g

Cauliflower Mash

Yields: 2 servings

Prep time: 5 minutes

Cook time: 10 minutes

Total time: 15 minutes

Ingredients

¼ cup of sour cream

½ head cauliflower

Salt and pepper

Directions

Trim your cauliflower head then cut into bite sized florets.

Fill a pot with a half inch of water to boil then reduce flame to steam and simmer the florets in a steam basket covered with a tight fitting lid until easily pierced with a fork; this should take about 10 minutes.

Drain the water from the pot leaving the cauliflower behind then season with pepper and salt.

Add in the sour cream (or if you like you can use 2 tablespoons of heavy cream and butter). Yogurt is also a good option.

Blend the florets using an immersion blender until they are creamy and fluffy

Dress with any mix-ins you want. You can try ham & cheddar, olives & feta and mushrooms & tarragon

Nutritional information per serving: Calories 85, Proteins 3g, Carbs 3g and Fats 5g

Peanut Butter Cookies

Yields: 15 servings

Prep time: 10 minutes

Cook time: 15 minutes

Total time: 25 minutes

Ingredients

½ cup of erythritol natural sweetener

1 egg

1 cup of peanut butter

Directions

Preheat your oven to 350 degrees F.

Combine the 3 ingredients in a mixing bowl.

Roll the mixture into 15 one-inch sized cookies then place on a baking sheet lined with silicone mat or parchment paper. Press down on the tops of the cookies using a fork.

Bake for about 10-13 minutes at 350 degrees F.

Allow the cookies to cool before serving. Store any leftovers in an airtight container.

Nutritional information per serving: Calories 117, Proteins 4g, Carbs 3g and Fats 9g

Low Carb Chicken Nuggets

Yields: 6 servings

Prep Time: 5 minutes

Cook Time: 13 minutes

Total Time: 20 minutes

Ingredients

1 teaspoon of garlic salt

¼ cup of almond flour

1 egg

8 ounces of cream cheese

2 cups of cooked chicken

Directions

Using an electric mixer shred the cooked chicken. If using leftover chicken, you need to warm it a bit. Add in the remaining ingredients once the chicken is shredded and mix until combined thoroughly.

Drop scoops of the mixture onto a lined or greased baking sheet then flatten into a nugget shape.

Bake for 12-14 minutes at 350 degrees F until firm and slightly golden.

Reheat frozen leftovers in the oven or toaster oven for about 10 minutes at 350 degrees or in the microwave for about 45 seconds.

Nutritional information per serving: Calories 243, Proteins 18g, Carbs 2g and Fats 17g

Keto Eggs

Yields: 6 servings

Prep time: 10 minutes

Cook time: 15 minutes

Total time: 25 minutes

Ingredients

4 oz. cooked bacon

12 eggs

Salt and pepper, to taste

Directions

Preheat your oven to 400 degrees F.

Line your muffin tin with cupcake liners – even if the surface is nonstick, you need to line it as eggs easily stick except if using silicon forms.

Crack one egg into each form then add in any Keto-friendly filling of choice – you can invent your own or choose one of the suggested fillings below. This recipe uses classic crumbled bacon

Season to taste then bake in the oven until the eggs are cooked; this should take about 15minutes

Filling suggestions

Salami, turkey, ham, all kinds of cheeses (e.g. parmesan, pepper jack, blue cheese) plus minced garlic, chopped onion, tomatoes, avocado and pickled or fresh jalapenos/chili pepper

Nutritional information per serving: Calories 205, Proteins 13g, Carbs 1g and Fats 16g

Spicy Roasted Nuts

Yields: 6 servings

Prep time: 5 minutes

Cook time: 10 minutes

Total time: 15 minutes

Ingredients

1 teaspoon of chili powder or paprika powder

8 oz. pecans or walnuts or almonds

1 teaspoon of ground cumin

1 tablespoon of coconut oil or olive oil

1 teaspoon of salt

Directions

In a medium frying pan, mix all ingredients then cook over medium heat until the nuts (this recipe used almonds) are warmed through.

Allow the almonds to cool before serving. Serve with a drink.

Store any leftovers at room temperature in a container secured with a lid.

Nutritional information per serving: Calories 285, Proteins 4g, Carbs 2g and Fats 30g

Conclusion

We have come to the end of the book. Thank you for reading and congratulations for reading until the end.

I hope this book has given you enough variety on the foods you can prepare to turn your body into the efficient fat burning machine that you want it to become using only five ingredients or less and yield only five net carbs or less.

If you found the book valuable, can you recommend it to others? One way to do that is to post a review on Amazon.

Click here to leave a review for this book on Amazon!

Thank you and good luck!

www.ingramcontent.com/pod-product-compliance
Lightning Source LLC
Chambersburg PA
CBHW021441210526
45463CB00002B/599